The Pocket
Handbook
of
Juice Power

Keats Titles of Related Interest

The Pocket Handbook of Juice Power

CARLSON WADE

Foreword by
Ray C. Wunderlich, Jr., M.D.

Keats Publishing, Inc. New Canaan, Connecticut

The Pocket Handbook of Juice Power is not intended as medical advice. Its intention is solely informational and educational. Please consult a medical or health professional should the need for one be indicated.

THE POCKET HANDBOOK OF JUICE POWER

Library of Congress Cataloging-in-Publication Data

Wade, Carlson.
    The Pocket Handbook of Juice Power / Carlson Wade : foreword by Ray C. Wunderluch.
        p. 96 cm.
    ISBN 0-87983-591-5 : $3.95
    1. Fruit juices—Health aspects. 2. Vegetable juices—Health aspects. I. Title.
RA784.W257   1992
613.2′6—dc20   92-19923
                                                     CIP

ISBN: 0-87983-591-5

Printed in the United States of America

Keats Publishing, Inc.
27 Pine Street (Box 876)
New Canaan, Connecticut 06840-0876

Contents

Foreword

RAY C. WUNDERLICH, JR., M.D.

Raw juices will never replace sex, or even watching a good movie. But the use of raw juices can enhance the former and enable the individual to enjoy the latter for many good years.

Few today disagree with the notion that health is related to diet. The knowledge that raw juices have special nutritive value, however, is not as widespread. The nutritional benefits of raw juices are most evident in those persons who are nutrient-deprived. The accumulated impact of convenience eating has taken its toll, and excessive use of antibiotics, birth control pills and corticosteroid drugs, along with the excessive consumption of fats, salt, sugar-coated and overcooked foods and undesirable food additives are associated with an epidemic of functional gastroenteropathy—faulty bowel function. It is unusual to find an individual over forty years of age who digests and absorbs his food properly and meets his nutrient needs from diet alone. Furthermore, the highly toxic nature of the environment poses the question of just how much undernourishment one can tolerate before succumbing to degenerative disease of one sort or another.

Given so many persons with faulty bowel function, it is no wonder that raw-juice therapy can produce such consistent beneficial effects. Raw juice makes almost no demand upon digestive organs struggling with a daily load of cooked and often devitalized junk foods. Raw juices are digested in a matter of minutes. Whole food—even good whole food—requires hours of gut work for digestion. So raw juices spare the gut and tend to restore or preserve body vitality.

Juices, though, do lack fiber, a dietary essential, so should not be relied on over prolonged periods to supply the whole of the body's nutrient needs. Fresh, whole, fiber-rich food is an important constituent of basic nutrient input. Additional fiber supplements may be needed during juice therapy.

Much of the value attributed to raw juice probably stems from the presence of raw enzymes. Cooked food lacks raw enzymes because food enzymes are inactivated by temperatures in excess of 130°F. Nature has apparently placed enzymes in raw foods to assist in the digestive process, relieving the food consumer of some digestive burden. Persons who utilize raw foods in their diets often experience increased energy. Some believe that additional benefits accrue because raw enzymes are absorbed by the blood and are used in other metabolic processes. If such is the case, not only the digestive organs but the tissues of the entire body may benefit.

When we arrive in this world we are meant to be fed with an enzyme-rich, easily digested ''raw juice''—breast milk. Throughout our lives we can benefit by the use of raw juices. Although there are some cases in which a professional may countermand their use, by and large we build health and forestall disease through consumption of this readily-absorbed, enzyme-rich food source—raw juices.

Introduction

To enjoy abundant health, you need to nourish your body with wholesome nutrients as created by Nature. Unspoiled by chemicals, spared the destructive effects of cooking, raw fruit and vegetable juices are rich concentrations of pure elements your body uses to build and rebuild your trillions of cells from head to toe.

Fresh juices easily prepared at home with your extractor are prime sources of vitamins, minerals, enzymes, carbohydrates, proteins, trace elements and many other nutrient treasures that will help repair the damaging results of harmful living habits.

You have been assaulted to one degree or another by injurious factors such as foods that are chemically poisoned, overcooked, refined or highly processed. You also face the problem of air pollution, water pollution and depletion of the planet's ozone layer with the risk that brings destructive rays and radiation. Add smoke, benzene, detergent, chemicalized dyes or cosmetics that seep through your body pores to wreak internal emotional and physical havoc. Toxic drugs or patent medicines join physical trauma to create a constant threat to your well-being.

How can you shield yourself from these enemies that seem to surround you wherever you live? One answer is to rebuild your immune system with richly concentrated nutrients as found in fresh raw fruit and vegetable juices. These elements provide a barrier to strengthen your resistance to the threat of bacterial and viral invaders that might otherwise break down your immune system and predispose you to endless ailments. These include respiratory problems, cardiovascular ailments, stress-related conditions, premature old age, skin and hair injury, loss of vital senses such as hearing and eyesight and taste, and reduction in the function of important body organs such as the liver, kidneys and gallbladder.

With the use of richly concentrated juices, a powerhouse of nutrients as created by Nature and untouched by processing, your immune system will be strengthened and invigorated to resist and cast out hurtful invaders and shield you against ill health.

Fresh raw juices are a Fountain of Youth to restore health and extend your prime of life—to help you feel forever young, forever healthy!

The Pocket
Handbook
of
Juice Power

1. The "Missing Link" Found in Raw Juices

Why should you drink instead of eat raw fruits and vegetables? The answer is that you should do both—but you need to drink a sufficient amount of fresh juices daily to provide your body with a "missing link" hard to obtain from the produce itself.

This life-giving element is needed for your survival—and, as well, it promotes your recovery from daily assaults by the environment and determines your degree of rejuvenation and feeling of total health. This element is found largely in fresh raw juices.

Meet Life-Giving Enzymes

Your body is made up of trillions of microscopic cells. Your very existence depends upon healthy cells. They require nourishment—*living* nourishment to give you *living* health. Your cells depend upon—enzymes!

The biochemical miracle that nourishes your

body, that gives you vitality and energy, is found deep within the structure of fruits and vegetables.

Enzymes are complex proteins which help you digest food and absorb it via your bloodstream, dispatching nutrients to every part of your body.

Enzymes are more than substances. They possess a vital energy which is essential to the action and activity of every part of your body, in fact, in every part of every life form, whether animal or vegetable.

Without enzymes there would be no life!

Cooked Foods vs. Raw Foods. You may know that when you cook food, you destroy various vitamins and minerals—but you're also destroying precious enzymes. Heating above 118°F. causes them to become weak and unable to perform their life-giving functions. Heating above 130°F., as in cooking, even for a short time, will kill the enzymes stone dead—and while the food you eat will have some nourishment, it will be entirely depleted of these life-giving elements.

Fruits and vegetables and grains and seeds are rich sources of enzymes—but ONLY when they are raw. Dormant enzymes in seeds under proper conditions can remain in suspended animation for hundreds of centuries—but even such handy enzymes survive and thrive only if spared cooking!

Enzymes, Digestion, Total Body Health. When you chew foods, then swallow, your digestive system uses enzymes to remove vitamins, minerals, amino acids and other substances to be sent via your bloodstream throughout your body for building and rebuilding your health.

Without enzymes, the food would remain in your stomach as a solid mass! It would not be broken down or assimilated. If you have a depleted enzyme supply, you experience only partial metabolic reaction and, obviously, partial healing throughout your body. Enzymes are catalysts in your system. They create the biochemical change of metabolism but do not become part of that change. After finishing their work, they retreat into your cells and await the next call to transform the food you've eaten into health-building elements.

A certain number of enzymes are used up or destroyed in the process, so that you need a steady daily supply to meet the requirements of around-the-clock metabolism.

Whole Foods or Juiced Foods? Whole fruits and vegetables that you chew thoroughly are, of course, the mainstay of life. Yet many folks chew improperly or have dental disorders that make it difficult or impossible to fully chew and withdraw the enzymes from whole fruits and vegetables. Your body receives only a partial supply of enzymes from such improperly chewed produce.

Fresh raw juices are a richly concentrated source of enzymes along with other nutrients. When you use an electric-powered or strong hand-powered extractor, the blades break down the tough fibrous connective tissues and "veins" found in many raw fruits and especially in green vegetables. The centrifugal action of the sharp blades will cut right through the woody exterior of the produce to release the enzymes and nutrients into the juice you drink.

Even if you have excellent chewing ability, it is difficult to break through the fibrous interior of many plant foods and the enzymes remain locked within, to be passed out with the undigested matter during the eliminative process.

With fresh raw juices, you break through the toughest of barriers as the whirring blades of the extractor penetrate and release an outpouring of these life-giving elements. These fresh juices are, obviously, uncooked and therein lies their power, since enzymes have not been depleted or destroyed as they would when subjected to cooking, processing or preserving with chemicals. You DRINK the rich powerhouse of ALL the life-giving substances in the produce as put there by Nature. You receive total nutrition from whole foods that have been made liquid in a matter of moments.

How Raw Juices Rebuild Health

Enzymes in raw juice are speedily used to promote healing and regenerative processes. They improve your digestive functions, they participate in assimilation and elimination.

A raw juice will help break down other nutrients into simple substances that can be rapidly absorbed into the bloodstream. The enzymes in the juices easily perform these difficult biological processes

The "Missing Link" Found in Raw Juices

without heat and without themselves becoming part of the change. For this reason, they are called catalysts.

A variety of raw juices is used by the body to provide a continuous source of these enzymes. Each enzyme is specific; that is, it works upon one substance only. After its work has been finished, it is destroyed. You need to drink several glasses of freshly squeezed juices daily to have an adequate supply of enzymes and other nutrients available for inner healing.

For example, if you have been feeling sluggish, fatigued, without much energy, the remedy is to drink a glass of freshly squeezed orange juice. The powerhouse vitamin C will speedily supercharge you with energy and vitality in a matter of moments. The enzymes will use this vitamin C to repair broken or damaged cells and strengthen your inner structure so that you have more vigor and youthful vim. This is the power of a raw juice.

Another example: Your skin seems sallow and prematurely aged, and you are troubled with creases, wrinkles and sag. Drink a glass of freshly squeezed carrot juice. The rich supplies of enzymes and beta-carotene will soon make their way to your blood circulation to repair your skin from beneath its surface.

Let us go for one more benefit. You have difficulties with your bladder and kidneys. Drink a glass of freshly juiced yellow fruits such as cantaloupe, peaches, nectarines, papaya. You nourish your internal organs with a rich concentration of enzyme-powered vitamin A to help strengthen your membranes and detoxify your system of hurtful invaders. You build resistance to infections with the nutrients in a raw juice.

The enzymes found in raw whole foods and their juices are the "missing link" that connect you to the pathway to youthful health. You can drink your way to rejuvenation!

2. *Vitamins in Raw Juices*

Your body requires vitamins to help fight infection, initiate new cell growth, build a healthy skin, maintain a strong nervous system and to become involved in the metabolism of protein, fats and carbohydrates. You need vitamins on a daily basis since few of them are stored for future use.

Raw Juices or Whole Foods for Vitamins? The answer is to maintain a balance but tip the scales in favor of more raw juices. Basically, a rule of thumb is to eat cooked foods (particularly those that obviously cannot be eaten raw) but increase intake of fresh raw juices.

When you extract vitamins from fresh raw fruits and vegetables, you provide all body cells with the elements they need for speedy assimilation.

On the other hand, whole foods whether eaten raw or cooked will help you sustain life. But they do not have the concentrated power to regenerate the atoms which provide life forces to your body. To help protect against progressive degeneration of the cells and tissues through consumption of cooked and processed foods, boost your intake of vitamin-rich juices.

Fresh Is Best

All juices should be made fresh before using. If you must store juice, put it in a clean glass container, cover tightly and refrigerate promptly. Plan to use it within 24 hours for maximum nutritional benefit. Certain juices are especially rich in vitamins (among other nutrients) which have a positive effect on specific conditions, and go to work within 30 minutes to produce desired benefits. Here is a handy at-a-glance checklist of selected juices with super-vitamin power.

Vitamin A

Why It's Needed. Necessary to new cell growth. Helps fight infection. Essential for healthy skin, good blood, strong bones and teeth, kidneys, bladder, lungs and membranes. Seems to extend longevity. Does not occur as such in whole foods but as a provitamin, beta-carotene or carotene which is transformed by the body into vitamin A. Helps protect against cancer and enhances the immune system.

Raw Juice Sources. Carrots, spinach, tomatoes, green and red peppers, cabbage, celery, rose hips, oranges. TIP: absorption of vitamin A into your digestive tract is boosted by adding a bit of sesame seed oil to the juices, about one teaspoon per 10-ounce glass.

Vitamins in Raw Juices

Vitamin B1 (Thiamine)

Why It's Needed. Necessary for proper metabolism of sugar and starch to provide energy. Maintains a healthy nervous system and mental attitude. Stress increases the need for B1 and the other B-complex nutrients.

Raw Juice Sources. Grapefruit, carrots, beets, beet tops, spinach and dandelion; also found in brewer's yeast, wheat germ, bran, blackstrap molasses.

Vitamin B2 (Riboflavin)

Why It's Needed. Important to good muscle tone. Involved in metabolism of protein, fats and carbohydrates. Necessary for vision, skin, nails and hair health.

Raw Juice Sources. Parsley, turnip greens, carrots, beet tops, celery, green peppers, kale. Also in brewer's yeast.

Vitamin B3 (Niacin)

Why It's Needed. Involved in proper functioning of nervous system. Needed for healthy skin and good digestive system.

Raw Juice Sources. Parsley, kale, broccoli; also in brewer's yeast, wheat germ.

Vitamin B5 (Pantothenic Acid)

Why It's Needed. Helps form certain hormones and antibodies. Aids resistance to stress. Plays an essential role in energy, metabolism. Needed for maintenance of healthy digestive tract, skin and nerves and glands.

Raw Juice Sources. Cabbage, cauliflower, strawberries, grapefruit, oranges; also in brewer's yeast.

Vitamin B6 (Pyridoxine)

Why It's Needed. Essential for utilization of proteins and fats. Needed for production of red blood cells and antibodies to fight disease. Helps in normal functioning of nervous system. Natural diuretic, helpful for PMS.

Raw Juice Sources. Pears, lemons, carrots, bananas, green leafy vegetables; also in wheat germ and pecans.

Vitamin B12 (Cyanocobalamin)

Why It's Needed. Functions in coenzymes involved in nucleic acid synthesis and biological methylation. Assists in development of normal red blood cells and maintenance of nerve tissue.

Raw Juice Sources. Black currants, citrus fruits,

green peppers, kale, cabbage, parsley and rose
hips.

Folic Acid

Why It's Needed. Functions as part of coenzymes in amino acid and nucleoprotein metabolism. Forms red blood cells. A must for pregnant
women or those taking oral contraceptives.

Raw Juice Sources. Parsley, carrots, oranges,
potatoes, green leafy vegetables.

Biotin

Why It's Needed. Functions as part of a coen-
zyme involved in fat synthesis, amino acid metabolism and glycogen formation. May be essential
for biosynthesis of folic acid.

Raw Juice Sources. Cauliflower, lettuce, grapefruit; also in brewer's yeast.

Vitamin C

Why It's Needed. Helps hold body cells together; important in tooth, bone and blood formation, in healing of wounds, for health of adrenal
glands. Forms cementing substances such as collagen. Aids in use of iron. Helps resist infection,
colds and flu.

Raw Juice Sources. Broccoli, sweet and hot
peppers, collards, Brussels sprouts, strawberries,

orange, kale, grapefruit, figs, papaya, mango, tangerine, tomato, green leafy vegetables.

Vitamin E

Why It's Needed. An antioxidant that prevents premature oxygen reaction in the body; essential to use of oxygen by muscles. Prolongs life of red blood cells. Protects lungs; inhibits blood clot formation, prevents cell-membrane damage.

Raw Juice Sources. Green, leafy vegetables; also found in cold-pressed vegetable oils, especially wheat germ oil.

Vitamin K

Why It's Needed. Necessary for formation of prothrombin needed for blood clotting. Essential for normal liver functioning; important in maintaining vitality and longevity.

Raw Juice Sources. Alfalfa, green plants, leafy green vegetables, cabbage, carrot tops; also in blackstrap molasses and polyunsaturated oils.

Choline

Why It's Needed. Aids in nerve transmission and utilization of fat. Helps prevent fat deposits in liver and degenerative changes in kidney and bladder.

Raw Juice Sources. Green leafy vegetables; also

found in brewer's yeast, wheat germ and especially lecithin.

Bioflavonoids (Rutin, Hesperidin)

Why They're Needed. Part of the vitamin C complex family. Protects strength of vitamin C and improves cellular integrity.

Raw Juice Sources. Lemons, grapes, plums, grapefruit, cherries, especially the stringy portion of the interior. Also in buckwheat.

3. *Minerals in Raw Juices*

Your body needs minerals to help build strong bones and teeth, to calm your nerves, to stabilize normal blood clotting effect and to participate in glandular actions.

Minerals are important in the formation of the skeletal structure, the maintenance of an acid-base balance, as enzyme catalysts (helpers) in biological reactions, as regulators of muscle contractility, as transmitters of nerve impulses and in the promotion of growth.

Caution: Minerals in Processed Foods Are Altered. Processing often dramatically changes the mineral format in most foods. There are some products that are so imbalanced that the end result is a food excessively high in sodium and depleted of other substances. Fresh, raw juices provide you with a beverage rich in minerals as created by Nature for much better assimilation and utilization in your body.

Here is a checklist of the valuable minerals and how to use them in juice form for specific needs.

Minerals in Raw Juices

Calcium

Why It's Needed. Works with phosphorus to build and maintain bones and teeth. Also works with vitamin D. Aids in blood clotting and important for nerve, muscle and heart function.

Raw Juice Sources. Deep green leafy vegetables, collards, dandelions, kale, mustard and turnip greens, broccoli and figs.

Copper

Why It's Needed. Assists in the formation of hemoglobin and red blood cells. Necessary for proper bone formation and production of RNA, the carrier of the genetic code. Involved in oxidation systems of the body.

Raw Juice Sources. Raisins, grapes, onions, almonds, green leafy vegetables.

Iodine

Why It's Needed. Essential component of thyroid hormone thyroxin which controls cell oxidation rate. (Goiter is a result of iodine deficiency.)

Raw Juice Sources. Oranges, spinach.

Iron

Why It's Needed. Combines with protein to build red blood cells which carry oxygen to all parts of the body. Critical in formation of hemoglobin. Absorption and proper utilization appears to be enhanced by vitamin C and copper.

Raw Juice Sources. Dark leafy green vegetables; sundried fruits such as apricots, figs, papaya, red and black currants; raspberries, parsley, beet tops.

Magnesium

Why It's Needed. Contributes to the health of nerves and muscles. Works with calcium and phosphorus to build and maintain bones and soft tissue; activates enzymes for carbohydrate metabolism; contributes to formation of body proteins, maintenance of body temperature, muscle contraction and nerve impulse transmission.

Raw Juice Sources. Elderberries, raspberries, lemons, beets, figs, nuts, dates, citrus fruits, leafy greens.

Manganese

Why It's Needed. Involved in the reproductive process. Activates enzymes related to carbohydrate, protein and fat metabolism. Promotes normal bone structure.

Raw Juice Sources. Strawberries, apricots, oranges, greens such as lettuce and kale, figs, watercress.

Phosphorus

Why It's Needed. Builds bone and teeth in combination with calcium and vitamin D. Preserves acid-alkaline balance. Critical to every body cell as an essential factor in protoplasm. Aids in transformation of chemical energy into body reactions and in metabolism of carbohydrates; fosters feelings of energy.

Raw Juice Sources. Grapes, raspberries, tangerines, carrots, cabbage, beet tops, watercress, kale, figs.

Potassium

Why It's Needed. Works with sodium to maintain cell fluid balance; establishes electrical potential to permit healthy nerve impulse conduction. Works with magnesium to utilize amino acids. Works with calcium to maintain nerves. Helps muscles contract and aids in carbohydrate metabolism.

Raw Juice Sources. Grapes, tangerines, lemons, parsley, potatoes, dandelions, celery, kale, tomatoes, bananas, mushrooms.

Selenium

Why It's Needed. Nourishes each and every cell of the body. Believed to resist and protect against certain types of cancer. As an antioxidant, fights off and "defuses" harmful free radicals. Also said to help slow down the aging process. Acts as a "cleanser" to sweep out potentially dangerous viral and bacterial invaders.

Raw Juice Sources. Carrots, cabbage, cauliflower, garlic, green pepper, lettuce, mushroom, onion, radishes, tomatoes, apples, bananas, oranges, peach, pear, pineapple.

Zinc

Why It's Needed. Participates in many cell activities involving proteins, enzymes, hormones, wound healing, normal growth. Makes up part of the enzyme necessary for carbon dioxide transport; an essential component of the pancreatic insulin hormone. Believed helpful for problems of the reproductive organs, especially, in men, the prostate gland.

Raw Juice Sources. Green leafy vegetables, fruits, garlic; also found in brewer's yeast, pumpkin seeds.

To boost your basic health, include an ample supply of minerals via raw juices. Often overshadowed by vitamins, minerals may well be just as vital or more so in your quest for a healthy body and mind.

4. *Super-Protein from Raw Juices*

We hear much these days about a high-protein diet for the basics of health. Perhaps "high-quality protein" would be more appropriate to the body's needs. This is available to you, first-hand, through the use of raw juices from meatless sources.

Limits of Cooked Protein. Protein is abundant in animal products such as meat, fish, poultry, eggs, dairy products. These, obviously, need to be cooked in order to be eaten or, in the case of dairy products, they are first processed and packaged. When you eat cooked protein, only about one-third is made available to the body. The other two-thirds are taken up by the body to be disposed of (which also takes much effort and energy) in due time. If you have ever felt sleepy after eating an animal food, you now know that it's because of the metabolic requirements that follow.

The Protein Pathway to Digestion. The cooked protein you eat must be split up into amino acids to get through the membrane walls of your alimentary canal. Proteins as such are not readily diffusable. A problem is that if your digestive system cannot completely break down the proteins, you could develop allergic reactions.

If your digestive tract or alimentary canal becomes overloaded with a partially-digested mass of protein material, toxic wastes are released through decomposition. These harmful wastes have been implicated in many illnesses, notably colon cancer. So it becomes evident that protein digestion is of more health-building value than protein intake quantity.

In brief, the primary function of protein in the diet is to supply the materials—amino acids—which are utilized by your body to build and rebuild tissues. Dietary proteins must first be split into their constituent amino acids before they can be absorbed by your bloodstream. Blood then carries amino acids to the tissues which, in turn, select the kinds and amounts of amino acids needed for the particular protein synthesis.

Essential Amino Acids. Of approximately 20 amino acids utilized in the synthesis of proteins, eight are known as "essential" because they cannot be made in your body by other substances and must come from foods.

Nonessential Amino Acids. If this group is missing from the diet, they may be biosynthesized by your body from metabolic products of other nutrients.

Benefits of Protein. In addition to building new tissues during the growth process, proteins are needed for the maintenance of existing tissues. A dynamic equilibrium exists between the proteins in the cells and the amino acids dispatched via food digestion.

Proteins have necessary regulatory functions in your body. If the protein level in blood is low, extra water is drawn into the tissues and edema (water retention) results. Proteins also are involved in the systems regulating the acid-base balance which maintains acidity of body fluids at the required level. You must keep your acid level within narrow ranges to sustain life.

Proteins are also constituents of important hormones and enzymes which are involved in a variety of metabolic body processes. Life is protein!

Cooked vs. Raw Protein

Protein from familiar sources such as meat, eggs, dairy products and seafood may be correctly identified as "complete" protein containing all essential amino acids. But—cooking and processing destroys some, if not all, of many of these "essential" amino acids and this distorts the pattern. Most cooked proteins could then become incomplete.

Raw protein is found in foods that do not require cooking and may be considered "incomplete," but actually offer more than cooked protein. For example, nuts, seeds, avocados and whole grains may be combined with raw leafy vegetables in a juice to give you a complete amino acid pattern easily assimilated and more thoroughly digested by the body.

Drink Raw Protein Juices. In your juice extractor, you can combine a variety of nuts and seeds with raw greens to create a complete protein drink. Since you drink the juice made from raw foods, you have a complete amino acid pattern, along with valuable vitamins, minerals and enzymes.

Putting More Protein into Raw Juices

Excellent sources of protein will be found in brewer's yeast, wheat germ, lecithin, whole grains. Whenever you make a raw fruit or vegetable drink, add one or two teaspoons of these grains before you start the extractor. Within moments, you will have a protein-packed raw juice drink your body can handle without any waste residue left behind, as is the case with animal protein.

Easy-to-Make Protein Raw Juices

To have a complete amino acid pattern, try these recipes in your juice extractor:

- Raw assorted greens with cashews or other nuts.
- Various greens with sprouted seeds or grains.
- Combine your green beverage with nonfat cottage cheese.
- Add nonfat yogurt to any fruit or vegetable drink.

Enjoy these protein-packed (vitamin- and miner-

Super-Protein from Raw Juices

al-packed, too) raw juices and nourish your body
with much-needed nutrients.

High-Protein (No-Cow) Milk Drink

1 cup assorted nuts or seeds
1 cup cool water
2 teaspoons honey
½ teaspoon soy milk powder
  sprinkle of sesame seeds
2 California figs (very high in fruit calcium and
  protein)

Place everything in your extractor bowl. Buzz
for one to two minutes. The outpouring is milk
that is rich in meatless protein along with an abundance of vitamins, minerals and enzymes. (The
combination of nuts—especially cashew—with the
sesame seeds and figs gives a cow's milk flavor.
You could also try sunflower seeds for an exciting
milk flavor and taste.)

Go for the Balance

You can appreciate the importance of raw juices
for protein as against cooked animal protein. Heat
not only destroys enzymes and water-soluble vitamins, but makes some of the amino acids unavail-
able by forming linkages which your digestive
system cannot split. A good idea is to aim for a
balance—obtain raw-food protein from your juices
and, if you wish, get some animal-source protein
from cooked foods.

5. *Super-Health Green Drinks*

When you look at vegetables, you see the green leaves and wonder what they contain to make them so important.

They are full of life—ready to impart their precious heritage to your body, too.

All of life's energy comes from the sun. Green plants are in harmony with solar energy and use it to enrich and nourish all who eat whole foods grown from the soil. Chlorophyll, the green coloring matter used by Nature to color the woods, fields and forests as well as gardens, may be compared to hemoglobin, the red pigment in blood.

Hemoglobin consists of carbon, hydrogen, oxygen and nitrogen atoms. All are grouped around one iron atom. The pigment in green leaves is identical except that the central atom is magnesium. This near-identity of human and plant "blood" makes green leaves a source of vibrant health—available to us through raw juices.

Cooked Foods Have Limitations. While it is true that cooked and processed foods may sustain life, they do not have the ability to regenerate the atoms which furnish the life force to your body. In fact, they can contribute to the gradual deterioration of the cells and tissues. Deplete or deny your body enzymes and other nutrients through raw foods and juices and you may well see your health slipping through your fingers, a little at a time.

Invigorating Benefits of Green Leaf Juices

Plan to enjoy at least two or three glasses of freshly squeezed raw juices made from a variety of freshly washed green-leafed vegetables. The rewards:

1. Since they are raw, they pick up and utilize life-giving enzymes.

2. Green leaves are a prime source of vitamins, minerals and other nutrients that are quickly assimilated by your body.

3. Green leaf juices will have important amino acids when you use them in combination. Add a handful of nuts, sesame and sunflower seeds and you have a beverage whose protein power rivals that of animal foods.

4. Green juices have an alkaline reaction in the body to help protect against acid buildup.

5. A glass of green juice will have as much as 70 to 80 percent organic water—quite a difference from that which you pour from your kitchen tap as it comes from a chemicalized reservoir. The purest and most natural water is found in a raw green juice drink.

6. Greens are a good source of bulk or fiber.

The unique reaction is that nutrients in the green juice will create a highly magnetized reaction while passing through the gastrointestinal system. The juice cleanses the body of its used-up tissues and cellular wastes. It detoxifies the system and acts as an intestinal broom, washing out wastes that could be potentially hurtful.

7. An overall bonus of a green juice is that its mineral and chlorophyll content will stimulate your bone marrow to manufacture hemoglobin. Your body enjoys improved ability to digest and utilize food. You will have more resistance to illness and aging. Green juices build your immune system to create a barrier against common and uncommon disorders.

The nutrients are released from the "coils" of the plant via juicing and your body receives them full force and without any interference of woody barriers. Green leaves are refreshing juices you can drink your way to better health.

How to Plan Your Raw Juice Program

How much should you drink? A rule of thumb that applies to almost anything is—drink comfortably without forcing yourself or upsetting yourself.

Some have reported that one quart of fresh raw juices daily will soon show results. You may drink several glasses in the morning, then at noontime and in late evening. You will thereby be giving your body (and mind) a steady supply of the valuable elements needed to improve health.

Super-Health Green Drinks

About Juicers

An electric juicer works effectively to release the nutrients from the microscopic cells of the interior of fruits and vegetables.

You may consider a centrifugal type of juice extractor which functions on the principle of a fast-rotating plate with a sharp grating surface at the bottom of the basket in the machine. The rotation is very fast. The pulp is grated on the bottom plate, then flung by centrifugal force against the sides of the perforated basket. The juice from the pulp is then separated and collected through a spout.

The very purpose of raw juices is to help your body assimilate all of the vital elements found in the whole food in the quickest and easiest manner. You do not want to overburden your digestive system with excessive work. That is why a juicer is so important, because by means of a thorough trituration or grinding, it will rip open the fibers in the food and draw out the needed nutrients that will give life to your body—as it has done for the plant.

A variety of different green-leafed plants that make up a raw juice help revitalize your entire being. Draw upon the life energy of the sun through a green juice!

See Chapter 7 for more on juicers.

6. Raw Juice Help for Common Ills

Fresh raw juices are powerhouses of rich concentrations of nutrients that help strengthen your immune system to initiate healing for many health setbacks. In some situations, several glasses of juices will help turn the tide against disturbing conditions. In others, you will be able to regenerate your body by following a regular daily program of raw juices. Since they are all natural, they may be enjoyed freely.

The following suggestions should be considered as general information and a guide for improving health with juices.

INFECTIOUS DISORDERS. Black currants, citrus fruits, pineapple, Hawaiian papaya, elderberries, beets, green and red peppers, garlic and rose hips.

GASTRIC UPSET. Carrots, tomatoes, celery, Hawaiian papaya, figs. Cabbage juice is believed especially soothing for ulcers and gastric catarrh.

LIVER UPSET. Grapes, carrots, beets, dandelion greens (small amounts), Hawaiian papaya, figs and radishes.

Raw Juice Help for Common Ills

GALLBLADDER PROBLEMS. Cool inflammation with pear juice combined with Hawaiian papaya juice.

CONSTIPATION. Figs, prunes, Hawaiian papaya, grapes, apples.

GAS DISORDERS. The juice of yellow onions mixed with carrots or celery. Use only one tablespoon of the onion juice with the larger amounts of the other vegetables.

CHRONIC IRREGULARITY. Figs, prunes, Hawaiian papaya, yellow onion juice (one tablespoon mixed with other juices), carrots, cucumber, tomatoes, celery.

UPSET STOMACH. Apple juice, lemon juice mixed with pear or Hawaiian papaya juice. Blueberry juice is effective in controlling diarrhea. TIP: steep tea from dried blueberries to ease diarrhea.

BLOODSTREAM. Enrich the rivers of your body with kale, parsley, grapes, beets, blueberries. Rich in iron and chlorophyll, they help improve the production of red blood cells. Also nourishing for the small capillaries.

HEART. Add a small amount of garlic juice or pressed liquid from hawthorn berries to a mild vegetable juice. Helps soothe the heart muscle.

BLOOD PRESSURE. Boost intake of calcium, potassium with figs, Hawaiian papaya, bananas and also a small amount of garlic juice.

FATIGUE. Citrus fruits, black currants, grapes, pineapple, Hawaiian papaya, celery, beet and grape juices.

WATERLOGGED TISSUES. Also called edema, and often traced to sodium accumulation in the cells and tissues. Raw juices are very low in sodium. If possible, consider a raw juice fast for one or two days and help wash out the sodium from your system and your limbs, too. Fruit juices are especially low or free of sodium. Pear or dandelion juices are helpful.

LEG ULCERS or prominent varicose-like veins. Add garlic and onion juice to carrot juice. Helpful are apple juice and various citrus juices. TIP: to speed healing, use poultice made of cabbage or comfrey leaves.

OVERWEIGHT. Control your taste buds and appetite with juices from celery, parsley, citrus fruits, pineapple and grape juice. Hawaiian papaya is soothing and satisfying as an appetite suppressant. Small amounts of fig juice will also ease eating urges.

ARTHRITIC STIFFNESS. Juices are especially helpful in correcting metabolic errors responsible for rheumatic problems. Raw vegetable juices produce an alkaline action to dissolve the accumulation of deposits surrounding the joints. (Avoid tomatoes, peppers, potatoes.)

JOINT STIFFNESS. Improve the function of stiff joints with juices made from carrots, beets, alfalfa, celery and a small amount of parsley. Boost intake of raw vegetable juices since you want to correct the mineral imbalance in your tissues.

Raw Juice Help for Common Ills

BLOOD SUGAR. String beans, cucumber, celery, lettuces, citrus juices and some garlic juice. Boost intake of carbohydrate juices from most vegetables. Cucumber juice has a substance that revitalizes the pancreas to produce insulin to stabilize blood sugar. Onions contain a molecular cousin of sulfuric acid known as allinin, which is a powerful fungicide and even believed to be an antibiotic. It helps cleanse the system of accumulated wastes and also balances the blood sugar. One teaspoon of onion juice added to a glass of favorite raw vegetable juice will be adequate for most needs.

CARDIOVASCULAR DISORDERS. For stroke-like conditions, banana puree or juice provides much valuable potassium and vitamin B6.

DIABETES. Many have found that string beans contain trace minerals and important hormonal substances closely related to insulin. Raw bean juice in small amounts is regarded as helpful.

KIDNEY HEALTH. Small amounts of horseradish, with a squeeze of watercress and carrot and celery juices, are soothing. To help counteract uric acid in the bladder, small amounts of lemon juice in vegetable juices will be helpful.

PROSTATE GLAND. Add important vitamin E from a capsule or oil to a vegetable juice. Hawaiian papaya juice is regarded a helpful remedy for disorders of the prostate.

SKIN HEALTH. A day or two of raw juice fasting has been reported as healthful to the skin. In particular, citrus fruits are prime sources of ascorbic acid for speedy formation of collagen under the skin surface and improve basic health. Enjoy the colorful juices of grapes, carrots, beets, black currants, raspberries, strawberries. Fig juice is helpful for inner cleansing to remove toxins responsible for skin blemishes. Hawaiian papaya juice is a rich source of beta-carotene needed for skin health. Cucumber juice, with its rich mineral content, has long been used as a therapeutic help for skin problems.

NERVOUS DISORDERS. Fig juice is a rich source of calcium to help calm the nervous system. To induce sleep, try apples, carrots, oranges and celery.

BREATHING PROBLEMS. The raw juice of carrots, parsnip, potatoes with a sprig of watercress is soothing and helps clear away debris that cause problems. In particular, oranges, lemons, rose hips and a bit of garlic will make a healthful tonic. Breathe easier with grapefruit juice. A one- or two-day fasting program with citrus juices helps cleanse the respiratory tract.

ASTHMA. To rebuild the immune system so that you help resist sensitivity to irritants that could otherwise trigger a respiratory reaction. Dilute one tablespoon of plain lemon or lime juice in water first thing in the morning. Repeat several times throughout the day if you have recurring asthmatic problems. Take small amounts of garlic and carrot juices.

SKIN, NAILS, HAIR. Green pepper juice is a

prime source of silicon, which nourishes your body envelope. Combine with some carrot juice to help cleanse the system of toxic debris.

DIGESTIVE HELP. One speedy healer is Hawaiian papaya juice. When triturated and pressed, the extracted juice contains a principle known as papain. It has a similar effect to pepsin in the digestive process. It is also rich in fibrin, which corrects disorders of the digestive system. Papaya juice has also been found helpful in correcting intestinal disorders in a short time.

BLOOD VESSEL HEALTH. Raw parsley is a source of concentrated juice to be taken in small amounts (one or two ounces) in combination with other raw vegetables such as carrot, celery, lettuce. The parsley juice combines with the other vegetable juice to boost oxygen metabolism and maintain healthy action of the hormone network. Never drink too much raw parsley juice, even diluted, since its high concentration may result in disorders of the nervous system. A small amount goes a long way toward nourishing the capillaries.

HEART SAVER. Potassium is an important mineral needed to stabilize health of the heart. A potassium broth is easily made from the juice of carrots, celery, parsley. Drink regularly as a heart-saving tonic.

SKIN BLEMISHES. Raw potato juice has been found helpful in clearing up skin blemishes. A glass of potato juice has a high amount of sulphur, phosphorus, potassium and chlorine. The benefit here is that in the cooked potato, organic atoms become inorganic and there is a release of solanine (an alkaloid toxic substance) that could be distressing. Fresh raw potato juice is free of this reaction. Combine with carrot and celery and drink in moderate amounts to help cleanse the system of infectious irritants that could be responsible for skin disorders.

IMPROVED METABOLISM. Troubled by a sluggish circulation? Try fresh raw tomato juice with a squeeze of lemon or lime juice or even a squeeze of garlic juice. Tomato juice has a high citric and malic acid content which is beneficial for the metabolic process.

COLITIS. Cool off inflammation of the colon with the high mineral content of raw vegetable juices. Enjoy cucumber, lettuce, carrot, celery either singly or in combination.

Juice: Good for What Ails You

In general, natural medicine specialists and old wives alike agree that vegetable juices are necessary for building a strong body and regenerating its tissues, while fresh fruit juices act as cleansers and purifiers for bodily systems. Here's a brief rundown on some of both, and how and why these juices—in their fresh, raw states—have been used therapeutically to treat and prevent various ailments and conditions.

Berry Juice

Blueberries, huckleberries and strawberries act as natural astringents and blood purifiers. The first two are also natural antiseptics. Diabetics and those who suffer from menstrual problems can often benefit from berry juices, which are also very tasty for novices to juicing. Strawberries are excellent for clearing up skin conditions as well. Can't sleep? Try a soothing sipper made from elderberries before retiring. You'll sleep like a baby.

Brussels Sprout Juice

This juice is a delight—especially for diabetics who can benefit from the vast store of natural insulin within. Pancreas function is even more improved when starches and sugars are eliminated from the diet, and drinks of Brussels sprouts, string beans and lettuce are imbibed instead.

Cabbage Juice

The old school of thought for treating ulcers used to prescribe milk. Now that milk has been shown to aggravate, not heal, ulcers, researchers have returned to the roots of natural medicine for a real cure: raw, fresh cabbage. Try drinking a quart of cabbage juice a day, in small glassfuls five times throughout the day. Taken regularly, cabbage juice can apparently head off ulcers in those prone to them. Some people prefer to drink a mixture of fifty percent cabbage juice and fifty percent celery juice, which appears to have the same benefits.

Carrot Juice

Raw, fresh carrot juice is rich in vitamin A, also contains vitamins B, E and C, and acts as a normalizer on all the body systems. From one to as many as six pints of carrot juice may be taken each day—but cut back if your skin begins to turn orange! Carrot juice is especially beneficial to invalids or people recovering from illness because it boosts the appetite (try serving it as an appetizer) and aids digestion. Nursing mothers in particular benefit from carrot's crunch. In addition, carrots help to improve and maintain the bone structure of your teeth. And yes, a combination of carrots, celery and spinach will help keep your eyesight sharp and your eyes bright.

Celery Juice

Not all sodium is bad, and celery juice packs a lot of organic sodium in each glass you drink. This is especially useful in treating arthritis, particularly if all white flour, sugar and starch is eliminated from the diet for a time while you drink celery juice regularly. Combined with carrot juice, this healthful beverage helps cleanse the body of too much acid, and aids in tissue regeneration—including joint ligaments and the nervous system. (Disorders which result from the degeneration of the nerve sheath can often be relieved or alleviated with fresh carrot and celery juice, taken therapeutically.) Celery juice even soothes frazzled nerves and promotes restful sleep in chronic insomniacs.

Cherry Juice

Cherries act as alkalizers on the body and have a slight laxative effect, so you shouldn't drink too much of the concentrated juice at a time. Cherry juice is also soothing to nervous stomachs, boosts circulation, and is helpful to those with low blood pressure.

Cucumber Juice

Nature's diuretic! This juicy vegetable helps promote urination, and also grows hair, due to its rich silicon and sulphur content. Cukes are also very rich in potassium and phosphorus. Mix the juice with lettuce, spinach and carrots for a nutritional wallop. Cucumbers mixed with carrots help reduce uric acid in the body. (Add some beets to spur this combination on.) Reducing uric acid can help those with rheumatic ailments considerably.

Dandelion Juice

One of Mother Nature's most valuable minerals—magnesium—is right under your feet. Dandelion greens act as a powerful tonic, counteracting too much acidity and creating a normal alkalinity in the body. These weeds are also high in potassium, calcium and organic sodium. Magnesium helps prevent osteoporosis and prevents bone softening, especially in conjunction with calcium. Combine turnip and carrot leaves with dandelion greens for a real bone-booster. Dandelion juice is also a favorite in France, because of its beneficial action on the liver.

Garlic Juice

Aside from its reputed ability to vanquish vampires, garlic juice is very helpful in regulating high blood pressure. Its other heart-healthy effects include promoting better blood circulation and preventing arteriosclerosis.

Grape Juice

Drinking fresh grape juice is one of the best things you can do for your heart (assuming you don't smoke and haven't clogged your arteries with fat).

Green Pepper Juice

For strong, beautiful nails and hair, this is the juice to choose. Mix a small amount of it with carrot juice for the best results. Its effectiveness comes from the silicon content. Green pepper juice is also helpful in cases of colic, gas and even skin eruptions.

Kale Juice

Very rich in vitamin A, this green helped preserve the health of English citizens who ate kale in abundance during strict war-time rationing of most other foods. Iron, phosphorus, sulphur, potassium and calcium are all found in these health-giving leaves. One cup of kale provides as much as 37,000 IU of vitamin A, plus ample amounts of C, and riboflavin (a B vitamin).

Lemon Juice

Prone to colds and respiratory ailments? Pucker up! Lemons are pumped full of bioflavonoids, which help regulate body chemistry and play an important role in longevity and cell rejuvenation. But they are perhaps best known for their vitamin C content and action against colds and flu.

Lettuce Juice

Tired of munching on the same ol' salad? Try drinking it instead for a concentrated nutrition boost. Lettuce juice is very high in iron and magnesium and therein lies its effectiveness.

Onion Juice

Don't cry! Onion juice is an excellent blood purifier and natural germicide. Drink some when you feel a nose, sinus or throat infection coming on and you'll head it off at the pass. Insomnia, rheumatism and anxiety respond well to onions too.

Orange Juice

We all know oranges are rich in vitamins C, A and B. But they also act as blood cleansers, and help restore alkalinity to our often acid-overloaded body systems. Plus, orange juice is naturally sweet and light-tasting, making it a welcome addition to almost any vegetable or fruit juice cocktail.

Parsley Juice

If you suffer from kidney woes, parsley juice (mixed with other fresh, raw foods) should be on your menu almost every day. Combine it with carrot and celery juice for a real rejuvenating and restoring effect. Parsley juice is very potent alone and too much (more than a tablespoon or so) may overstimulate the nervous system. But taken with other veggies or fruits, it cleanses the kidneys and acts as an aid to the nervous system, the optic nerves and the nerves of the brain, keeping them sharp.

Pear Juice

Another natural kidney stimulant. Take some before bedtime so its excretory powers can do their trick overnight.

Pineapple Juice

This taste of the tropics is rich in potassium, chlorine, sodium, phosphorus, magnesium, sulphur, calcium, iron and iodine—all the essential minerals. Vitamins A, B, and C are also present in abundance in its raw, fresh state. Bromelin contained within this fragrant fruit is also an excellent tonic for the pancreas.

Potato Juice

Throw away your antacids and stomach remedies and drink spuds instead. Potatoes reduce the secretion of gastric acid, which eases acid stomachs and heartburn.

Radish Juice

Troubled by chronic sinus problems or allergies that clog up your head? Head for the radishes. Mixed with carrot juice (solo, radish is too strong, even for jalapeño fans) and including the radish tops, it helps soothe the mucous membranes and cleanses the body of excess mucus. Horseradish sauce is also excellent for the same effect, if your taste buds are hardy enough. Radishes are almost one-third potassium; and one-third sodium, magnesium and iron. That's a lot of nutrients from a little red plant. Best of all, this head-clearing cure causes absolutely no harm to delicate and irritated sinuses.

Spinach Juice

Popeye was right: The potent combination of sulphur and iron in raw spinach is a great energizer and strength-builder. Anemics should drink this regularly for their ''iron-poor'' blood. High in vitamins C and E, and also folic acid (something the typical American diet is notoriously deficient in, and which is especially important for pregnant women), spinach juice is also great for inner cleansing. In fact, raw spinach juice can cure virtually any case of constipation within days. Mix it with orange and lettuce or watercress juice for a tastier, lighter beverage.

Strawberry Juice

These sweet favorite fruits are not only appetizing, they are good for you as well. Their iron and fruit sugar content are natural aids in skin care, cleansing within as well as without. Strawberries are also excellent tonics for nerves and glands. If you suffer from acidosis, a sluggish liver, anemia, a blotchy or poor complexion, or constipation, add strawberries into your diet wherever possible.

String Bean Juice

Like Brussels sprouts, string beans are excellent for diabetics, and juicing them makes this therapy convenient. Try these vegetables in combination with string beans: carrots and spinach; carrots, celery, parsley; carrots, lettuce, and Brussels sprouts.

Tomato Juice

Brimming with good health, a glass of tomato juice promotes proper function of the pancreas by stimulating gastric juices. It is also a natural alkalizer. (In fact, it shouldn't be taken along with any starch or sugar, such as during a meal containing these types of foods, because they will negate its effect.) Tomatoes are also rich in all the vital elements needed to fight acidosis.

Turnip Leaf Juice

These green leaves are loaded with calcium, making them especially beneficial to those who can't (or prefer not to) get calcium from dairy foods. Kids who drink this juice have the toughest teeth around and strong bones. Combine turnip leaves with carrots and a few dandelion greens for a nutritional powerhouse. Turnip leaves also act as an alkalizer on the body, because of their abundant potassium. They also contain iron.

Watercress Juice

Forget fancy sandwiches and drink your watercress instead for concentrated good health benefits. Vitamins A, B, C, and E are present in these lovely leaves, and watercress is an aid in blood cell regeneration. It is also rich in these minerals: potassium, sulphur, calcium, sodium, chlorine, phosphorus, magnesium, iron and iodine. But, because these elements are acid-forming, watercress juice should also be mixed with carrot and celery juices. Use watercress in any juice you mix up for internal cleansing.

A Guide for Your Raw Juice Program

1. For top nutrient power, use raw juices as freshly prepared as possible.

Raw Juice Help for Common Ills

2. If you must store, do so in a glass container, tightly closed and promptly refrigerated. Use as soon afterward as possible.

3. Health stores have different types of electric juice extractors to suit individual needs. Follow the instructions that come with the juicer.

4. Make an effort to use very fresh raw fruits and vegetables. If at all possible, select those that are organically grown as available at many health stores and organic farms.

5. If you must use mass-produced produce, you need to minimize the risk of poisonous insecticides. Wash produce gently. Warm water with a mild detergent helps cleanse away much of the chemical sprays. Rinse well several times in gradually colder water. A final rinse and a brushing will make the produce more acceptable.

Fresh Raw Juices—Nectar of Nature!

Tap into the magical springs of vibrant health by enjoying the delicious beverages of Nature . . . made right at home!

Look younger, live longer and extend the prime of life with the sparkling freshness of raw juices! They are truly the elixir of life!

7. *How to Pick a Perfect Juicer*

Juicers are available through mail order, in appliance and department stores, and at your local health store. The latter may be your best bet if you want to see one in action first before deciding on what's right for you.

And, because the better ones are expensive, it pays to compare. Chances are, once you see how great making your own fresh juice is, you'll want to use it a lot. So get one that can stand up to a lot of heavy-duty use, not a cheap model that will bend or break the second week you use it.

The ideal juicer will make a maximum amount of juice from a given quantity of any material. The residue will be rather dry and can be added to salads, soups or gravies for fiber, or used as garden compost. (Try the fiber from fruit over ice cream or desserts.) Some juicers leave almost no residue, but the juices are very pulpy. It's a matter of personal taste.

But a juicer must also be convenient and easy to use for maximum benefit. And again, since they are expensive, you'll need to consider your purchase carefully. Here are some questions to ask to

How to Pick a Perfect Juicer

help you decide which of the products on the market is best for you:

• How does it work? There are two basic types of juicers. One works by using centrifugal action to press the food against cutters through a feeding hole. The solids remain in a basket or catcher and the juice comes out of a spigot. Only about a pint of juice is released before the solids must be emptied out.

The other type is a continuous-action machine. The juice comes out one side of a feeder after the produce goes through rotating cutters. Solids are released on the other side. Although convenient for making more juice at a time, these machines aren't as powerful at separating the juice from the fiber as centrifugal models, so the juice is pulpier.

• How easy is it to clean? Juicers must be cleaned meticulously after each use to prevent bacterial growth and protect the machine's parts. Try to assemble and take apart the model you're interested in. If it's too much trouble, you may not use it as much—and won't reap the benefits of fresh juice.

• What is it made of, and is there a warranty? Aluminum models are often less expensive, but some people prefer to stay away from aluminum utensils and containers. Stainless steel and hard plastic are often combined for a more durable unit.

The absolute minimum warranty you should settle for should be one year. But top of the line juicers are usually guaranteed for 10 years, so you get what you pay for.

• Is it versatile, and does that make any increased cost worthwhile? Some juicers chew up seeds, pits, skins and all, for maximum nutritional value. Some also can be used to make nut butters, sherbets, chop meat, grind grains into flour, make baby food, etc. However, having these options means nothing if you only plan on using it for glasses of juice.

Other things to consider are: noise level, amount of vibration, how much space the appliance takes up, as well as how many servings of juice you can expect from each use.

Juicers by Name

Here is some information on a wide variety of juicers, in no particular order:

CHAMPION—A powerful continuous extraction juicer which can grate produce into baby food, mill grains and act as a food processor. The pulp comes out one end while the juice comes out another. Fairly easy to clean, and very versatile, but expensive.

OMEGA (formerly the Olympic)—A centrifugal juicer. It makes about one quart of juice before you have to empty the basket. It's made in the U.S., is guaranteed for 10 years and is easy to clean. An optional citrus attachment lets you juice citrus without having to peel it.

How to Pick a Perfect Juicer

ACME JUICERATOR—This juicer is from Waring Products and is a centrifugal type, capable of making one quart of juice at a time and with less noise than a blender. There is a 10-year guarantee on this machine, which is made in America. The juicer runs well with little vibration. It uses paper filters which line the basket, making it easy to clean. The filters also help the Acme give a "cleaner" juice with less pulp. There is also an optional citrus attachment.

VITA-MIX—A continuous extraction model that juices and much more. It also mixes hot or cold soups, bread dough, grinds meat and makes ice cream and nut butters. There is a five-year guarantee on parts. The juice it makes is rather thick because there is no residue left. Expensive.

PHOENIX—This continuous-action juicer has a low to moderate noise level and makes a lot of juice at a time, juicing produce skin, pits and all. Some people may find the juice too pulpy, and prefer to strain it.

BRAUN—A centrifugal juicer that makes enough for two. It needs to be cleaned out after every pint or so of juice. One of the less expensive models. The resulting pulp is very dry.

MOULINEX—This juicer is also less expensive and smaller, for small households.

Tips for Getting the Most
From Your Juicer

Once you start doing your own juicing, you'll discover that the taste of no other canned, bottled or frozen product can compare. Apple juice that you make yourself is 200 percent better than any you've ever tasted.

Experimenting with various combinations of fruits and vegetables is fun. But here are a few things you should know before you throw everything but the kitchen sink into the juicer you've chosen.

- Dandelion leaves can be rather tough; use the smaller ones for better flavor and texture (although a good juicer can handle the biggest leaves easily).
- Dandelion and some other greens, such as endive or escarole and purslane, have a slightly bitter taste, so it's best to mix these in small amounts with other vegetables for juice.
- Some flavors will seem to intensify in juice, while others will be surprisingly delicate. Celery juice or soup, for example, is very light, and adding too many other tastes disguises the celery altogether. Peppers also taste delicate in a juice. Radishes, on the other hand, can add a lot of spice and zing to a juice—but may make it taste too hot for some palates. So

How to Pick a Perfect Juicer

watch your proportions of ingredients and experiment to obtain the "bouquet" you desire.

- Most produce tastes best at its freshest, ripest point, but there are a few exceptions. Pears, for example, taste much better when juiced while still hard and firm (unless you want pear purée, or baby food, for example).
- Of course, using every nutritious part of produce is a major plus of mixing your own fresh juice. But some parts may add a bitter taste to juice. There are some peels and seeds you should remove before juicing, including: the peel of bananas and oranges; melon rinds (watermelon, honey dew and cantalope); pineapple skin; and apple, orange and lemon seeds.
- Don't expect to love everything you make immediately—our taste buds have been numbed by oversweet and oversalted processed foods. There is nothing wrong with adding a bit of honey, maple or date sugar to sweeten up your juice, especially when it's new to you.
- Honeydew melons are sweeter, higher in calories and usually more expensive than cantaloupes.
- Red (such as watermelon) and yellow melons generally have more vitamin A than the white and green varieties.
- Cranberries juice best when they are all hard and firm. A few spongy, leaky ones can make the whole batch taste spoiled, so choose carefully.

The Pocket Handbook of Juice Power

- To get the most juice out of citrus fruits, pick the heavier, thin-skinned varieties. Avoid any that look wrinkled. Grapefruit, lemons and limes that feel heavy for their size offer the most juice for your money.
- Seedless grapes generally yield more juice than those with seeds.
- Use the taste test if you're not sure about whether a certain part of a vegetable or fruit will add bitterness to the juice. Just taste the seeds, peel, or whatever you're questioning. If it tastes bitter, discard it.
- If you are preparing vegetables for juice later in the day, especially if you are peeling or chopping them, put them in a bowl with ice water or leave them in the refrigerator in water so they don't dry out in the meantime. And of course, you can use the water in the recipe. (A squeeze of lemon juice also helps them taste fresher, even if you aren't going to juice them later, just serve them raw, cold and wet.)
- You can control the consistency of your juice in two ways. The first is by getting to know your juicer or food processor—the longer you process the food, usually the thinner it gets. Some juicers may require that you strain your juice first if you don't like it pulpy. Others will remove most of the pulp.

  The second way is with the types of vegetables and fruit you mix. Veggies such as cabbage, cucumbers, squash, watercress, lettuces, etc. have a lot of water inside of them and make for thinner, lighter mixtures. Fruits such as watermelons are very wet, whereas pears juice up frothy or thicker.

- Don't forget to add spices and fine herbs for more flavor. Try adding fresh ginger to carrot juice, or a dash of cinnamon, nutmeg, or whole cloves. There are dozens of varieties of pepper from all over the world. Experiment with fresh-ground peppercorns (of course, your juicer will grind them for you).

So keep these features in mind when you try different combinations for juice. There is no limit to the flavors and textures you can create—the only limit is in your imagination! (If you are trying something you feel is rather radical, however, you should probably just juice a small quantity to try first—in case the experiment is not to your liking.)

To Get You Started . . .

Here's a list of some ingredients for juices to get you going:

string and green beans	leek
Brussels sprouts	fenugreek sprouts
kale	parsnip
beetroot	alfalfa sprouts
asparagus	carrots
kohlrabi	pumpkin
parsley	cucumber

pineapple
onion
potato
apricot
peach
beet and beet greens
bean sprouts
orange
Jerusalem artichokes
tomato
tangerine
grapefruit
chervil
comfrey
figs
peppers
bananas
plums
watercress
papaya
apple
turnip
prunes
scallions
chard
broccoli
melon
cherries

lettuce
cauliflower
grapes
horseradish
turnip and turnip greens
berries
plantain
fennel
lime
currants
persimmon
rhubarb
lemon
mango
spinach
nettles
coconut
quince
pomegranate
collard greens
garlic
zucchini
celery
dandelion
radish and radish sprouts
wheatgrass
purslane

8. *Delicious Recipes to Try*

Part of the fun of having a juicer is the spontaneity and creativity it allows you. You really don't have to refer to a recipe book to concoct your own luscious beverages and meal replacements. But, for those who are new to the game and would like to taste some tried and true combinations, here are a number of "recipes" you can whip up in minutes at home—with the freshest of fruits and vegetables.

Again, all of the ingredients you put into your juicer should be organic whenever possible, and at least washed and rinsed very well to remove any traces of dirt or possible chemical contamination. Cranberries should be washed in hot water. Imported produce is likely to be sprayed several times and deserves even more attention. Scrub produce with a vegetable brush to remove any waxy coatings if your machine takes ingredients whole and unpeeled. Otherwise, peel as directed.

Fabulous Fruits

Many of these fruit juice combinations can also be made into frozen treats or ices. Check the directions that came with your juicer to see what they recommend.

Orange Strawberry Treat

1 dozen peeled seedless oranges
3 cups hulled strawberries

Juice and enjoy. Also try oranges with raspberries, blueberries, blackberries, you name it.

Ban-Apple Breakfast Drink

1 apple, cored
2 bananas, peeled if desired
2 tbsp. honey
2 tbsp. wheat germ
1 tbsp. brewer's yeast (optional)
1 cup ice
½ cup water or orange juice

Pink Pears with Appeal

4 bananas, peeled
4 pears, cored
3 cups hulled strawberries
¼ lemon, peeled
½ orange, peeled

Delicious Recipes to Try

Taste of the Tropics

2 mangoes, peeled and pitted
1 avocado, peeled and pitted
1 cantaloupe, peeled
1/2 to 3/4 lime, peeled
1/4 tsp. sea salt
pinch of cayenne pepper (optional)

Be careful when preparing—many people are allergic to mangoes, especially the peel.

Banapple-O

3 tart apples, cored
2 ripe bananas (yellow with black spots), peeled
5 oranges, peeled
dash of sugar or honey (optional)

This is particularly good if made as a semi-frozen treat.

Peachy Avocado

6 peaches, pitted
2 avocados, peeled and pitted
1/4 lemon, peeled
dash of sugar or honey to taste
1/2 tsp. sea salt
1 orange, peeled (optional)

Serve icy cold.

Tasty Melon Trio

3 cups cantaloupe
3 cups honeydew melon
3 cups watermelon
1 tbsp. lime juice
¹/₄ cup orange juice or half a peeled orange
3 ice cubes
¹/₈ tsp. salt (optional)

Mix thoroughly and strain if you like before drinking.

Sweet and Sour Tomato

1 lemon, peeled
1 pound cherry tomatoes
4 to 5 oranges, peeled and pitted
¹/₈ tsp. sea salt (optional)

Serve very cold! Excellent summer cooler.

Nonalcoholic Cocktails

Sometimes, when you're entertaining or for special occasions, you may want to serve something a little lighter. These delicious beverages can be mixed with seltzer, club soda or sparkling water for a little more zip—and the taste of an elegant cocktail or punch. Ice can also be added for a frozen slushy-type of drink. (Experiment with the amounts if you decide to serve one of these in a punch bowl or large pitcher.) And of course, you can also add the appropriate liquor if you wish.

Delicious Recipes to Try

Piña Colada

1 cup fresh pineapple, peeled and cored
1 banana, peeled
1/2 cup cream of coconut or grated coconut and
* cream*
3 cups ice

For a dessert-type drink, add vanilla ice cream or ice milk to the mixture, and a little more pineapple. A splash of orange juice is nice too.

Cucumbers à la Elsie

4 cups buttermilk
2 cucumbers, peeled
1/2 tsp. sea salt

Juice and serve over ice. Add some mint leaves or hot pepper for variety and extra flavor.

Bossy's Blueberries

6 cups blueberries
1 cup heavy cream, half-and-half or plain yogurt
1/4 lemon, peeled
2 tbsp. honey or sugar

You don't even need a juicer for this one—a blender makes a great smoothie.

Mint Surprise

6 grapefruits, peeled
fresh mint leaves, enough to make about 1 cup
* chopped mint*

Juice and drink. One peeled lime makes this extra tangy.

The Pocket Handbook of Juice Power

Fruit Smoothie

1 cup low-fat or skim milk
any fruit
1/2 tsp. vanilla extract
3 ice cubes

Bahama Mama

1/2 apple, cored and peeled if desired
1/2 mango, peeled and pitted
1 lime, peeled
1/2 pineapple, peeled and cored
1/2 banana, peeled
1 cup cherries, pitted (optional)
1 orange, peeled and pitted
1 cup strawberries, hulled
2 cups ice, or 1 cup water and 1 cup ice

Minty Hawaiian

1 orange, peeled and pitted
1/4 to 1/2 pineapple, peeled and cored
2 tbsp. sugar or 1 tbsp. honey (or less, to taste)
1 lemon, peeled
1 mint leaf
1/2 cup water or sparkling water or seltzer
2 cups ice

Delicious Recipes to Try

Bloody Mary on the Wagon
4 large tomatoes or 6 plum tomatoes
¼ beet
¼ onion
1 stalk celery
1 clove garlic (optional)
⅛ lemon, peeled
2 springs parsley or cilantro
⅛ hot or bell pepper
dash of hot pepper to taste, or tabasco sauce
½ cup water (to serve warm, use hot water)

Double Apple Delight
¼ pineapple, cored and peeled
1 apple, cored
¼ cup sugar or 2 tbsp. honey (optional)
1 cup ice
1 cup seltzer or sparkling water

Summer Sipper
4 cups watermelon (without the seeds)
1 lemon, peeled
1 tbsp. honey or sugar (optional)
1 cup ice

Green Champagne
3 stalks celery with leaves
2 cups pineapple
2 cups ice or 1 cup ice and 1 cup sparkling water

Honey, Do!

1 cup honeydew melon
1 orange, peeled and pitted
1 wedge lemon, peeled
1 cup ice

Tart and Tangy

1 grapefruit, peeled, with a little of the white zest
1/2 cup cranberries
1 1/2 cups water, sparkling water or seltzer
2 tbsp. honey

Orange-Banana Eye-Opener

1 orange, peeled and pitted
2 bananas, peeled
1 cup ice
1/2 sparkling water or seltzer

Taste of Tahiti

1 mango or papaya or banana (peeled and pitted)
1 1/4 cups milk
1/8 lemon, peeled
1/4 cup cream of coconut
handful of ice cubes
lemon-lime soda

Mix all of the ingredients together except the soda. Serve with a few splashes of soda, or mixed half-and-half with lemon-lime soda or sparkling flavored water.

Delicious Recipes to Try

Strawberry Daiquiri

6 oz. can frozen lemonade concentrate
10 oz. package frozen strawberries
8 oz. strawberry yogurt
splash of rum extract
2 tbsp. lime juice
2 cups ice

Lime Daiquiri

12 oz. can frozen limeade
splash of rum extract
2 cups ice

Banana Daiquiri

3 frozen bananas, peeled
splash of rum extract
2 cups ice

Peach Daiquiri

3 cups frozen, sliced peaches
splash of rum extract
2 cups ice

Fruit Smoothie

1/2 fresh pineapple, peeled and cored
1 orange, peeled and pitted
1/2 apple, cored
2 tbsp. honey
2 cups ice
1/2 sparkling water or seltzer

Pink Smoothie

$^1/_2$ fresh pineapple, peeled and cored
2 bananas, peeled
$^1/_2$ pint fresh strawberries, hulled
1 tbsp. honey (optional)
$^3/_4$ cup water, or $^1/_2$ cup water or seltzer with $^1/_4$
   cup grenadine syrup
2 cups ice

Raspberry-Lime Fizz

$1^1/_2$ cups fresh raspberries or 1 cup frozen
   raspberries
$^1/_2$ peeled lime
2 cups ice
1 $^1/_2$ cups sparkling water or seltzer

Cranberry Pick-Me-Up

2 cups cranberries
2 apples, cored
1 banana, peeled
2 tbsp. honey
1 tbsp. wheat germ

This is also good in a blender, if you peel the apple. For a thicker ''smoothie'' type of drink, add some plain yogurt and a couple of ice cubes to the mixture in the blender or juicer.

Delicious Recipes to Try

Pine-Orange Passion

2 oranges, peeled
¼ pineapple, cored and peeled
¼ lemon, peeled
1 tsp. honey (optional)

Stir in some wheat germ and brewer's yeast and you have a hearty breakfast drink. This can also be whipped up in a blender in a jiffy, if you use only the juices of the fruit instead of the whole fruit.

Red Refresher

½ pineapple, cored and peeled
12 strawberries
10 to 12 sprigs of watercress
1 to 2 radishes

Tomato Sour

2 tomatoes
½ cup sauerkraut
1 tsp. wheat germ
1 clove garlic (optional)

Orange-Papaya Punch

2 oranges, peeled
1 papaya, peeled and pitted
1 tsp. wheat germ
some coconut (optional)

Rich in potassium, this juice is great for that mid-afternoon slump or to jump-start your morning. Those with low blood sugar especially need potassium.

Peach Fuzz

1 to 2 peaches, pitted
½ pineapple, cored and peeled
1 tsp. brewer's yeast
½ cup skim milk or plain yogurt

Mango Mama!

1 mango, peeled and pitted
8 strawberries
2 limes, peeled
2 tbsp. honey (optional)
¼ pineapple, cored and peeled
mint leaf (optional, or as garnish)
2 cups ice

Add ½ cup sparkling water or ⅓ cup of light rum if desired.

Peachy Keen

1 to 2 peaches, pitted
¼ lemon, peeled
½ orange, peeled
ice, mint leaf (if desired)

Delicious Recipes to Try

Perky Papaya

1 papaya, peeled and pitted
3 oz. water
ice
3 oz. skim milk or plain yogurt

This drink is rich in vitamin A and is a natural energy booster.

Coconut Cocktail

½ coconut, hulled
1 tbsp. raw almonds
3 tbsp. soybeans (presoaked or canned)
½ pineapple, cored and peeled
2 tbsp. sunflower seeds
1 tsp. brewer's yeast

The protein in this tropical drink will keep you going a long time. Almonds are rich in potassium, calcium and phosphorus, as well as tasty.

Go Nuts!

½ pineapple, cored and peeled
1 to 2 tbsp. roasted peanuts, shelled
1 tsp. wheat germ
1 tsp. brewer's yeast
dash of sea salt (optional)

The Pocket Handbook of Juice Power

You Say Tomato

2 tomatoes
3 red radishes
dash of sea salt

Papaya Passion

2 papayas, peeled and seeded
1/4 cup coconut
passion fruit to taste
1 banana, peeled
6 to 10 strawberries
ice

Raspberry Rhubarb R&R

1/2 cup raspberries
1/3 cup rhubarb stalks
1 apple, cored
   Never use rhubarb leaves—they are poisonous.

Pears—Perfect!

6 pears, cored and peeled
2 lemons, peeled
2 tbsp. honey (or to taste)
ice or sparkling water (if desired)

Blueberry Smoothie

2 cups blueberries
1 apple, cored and peeled
1/4 lemon, peeled
1 1/2 cups plain yogurt or skim milk
1 tsp. vanilla or 1 vanilla bean
dash of nutmeg as a garnish on top

Delicious Recipes to Try

Spicy Peach Smoothie
4 peaches, peeled
1 apple, cored and peeled
1/4 lemon, peeled
1 1/2 cups plain yogurt or skim milk
dash of cinnamon

Vivacious Vegetable Drinks

Approximate amounts are given for these combinations. You may adjust them to your taste as you learn more about juicing and develop favorites.

Spicy Vegetable Cocktail
This can be made with your favorite blend of vegetables, or with tomatoes, to make a nonalcoholic Bloody Mary.

About 24 oz. vegetable or tomato juice
1/2 tbsp. Worcestershire sauce
1/2 tsp. sea salt
1/4 tsp. oregano
1/2 tsp. celery salt or 1 celery stalk
3 drops of hot pepper sauce or tabasco, or more,
*   to taste*

The Pocket Handbook of Juice Power

Green Apple

2 to 3 apples, cored (and peeled, if desired)
1 stalk celery
1/8 lemon wedge, peeled
1 cup ice

Eve's Apple-Carrot Drink

3 carrots
1 apple, cored
1 tsp. honey
1 whole clove or dash of ground cloves

Sizzle and Spice

3 radishes
1/2 red pepper
1/2 cucumber
1/2 beet
1/4 cup radish sprouts

Careful, this is a hot one! Fans of spicy food will love it, but it's not for the faint of heart—or faint of tastebuds.

Best Beetroot

1 beetroot
5 leaves Romaine lettuce
1/2 an orange, peeled and pitted
3 carrots

Delicious Recipes to Try

Weeds, Wet and Wild

1 cup sunflower greens
¹/₄ cup radish sprouts
¹/₄ cup alfalfa sprouts
2 stalks celery
¹/₂ green pepper
¹/₂ summer squash or zucchini
2 cups purslane
¹/₂ beetroot

Seven Greens Sipping Salad

Simply take equal proportions of:
   parsley
   chives
   dill
   green peppers
   watercress
Add *¹/₂ cup mint leaves*
¹/₄ cup coriander leaves
¹/₂ lemon, peeled and pitted
1 to 2 tsp. sea salt
1 to 2 cups water, according to thickness desired

To make a salad dressing instead of a juice, just skip the water and add some cold-pressed safflower or sunflower oil instead!

Popeye Pepper-Upper

spinach leaves
1 cucumber
2 carrots, plus greens (greens are optional)

Soups—Warm or Cool

Check any good cookbook for leek (vichyssoise) soup (use scallions if leeks are too expensive), borscht (cold beet soup) or gazpacho (cold tomato-salad soup). You'll find that making them in your juicer is even easier. But here are a few others to try you may not have thought of.

Garden Soup

This can be served warm or cool, or diluted with more water and less oil for a juice instead.

3 cucumbers
2 to 3 stalks of celery with leaves
2 green peppers
$^1/_2$ cup chives
$^1/_2$ cup water
1 tbsp. wine vinegar
$^1/_8$ cup olive oil (or other oil, according to your taste)
2 to 3 tsp. sea salt or celery salt

Garnish soup with a little sour cream or plain yogurt, grated carrots or beets for more color and flavor.

Yogurt-Tomato Refresher

1 pound tomatoes
$^1/_2$ cup plain yogurt
1 tsp. kelp (optional)

That's it!

Delicious Recipes to Try

Celery Soup

1 celery head plus leaves
2 cups milk
2 tsp. sea or celery salt

Soup-er Salad

This soup is rich in texture and flavor.
3 to 4 leaves of escarole
1 to 2 celery stalks
1 small onion, peeled
1 cucumber
2 large tomatoes
$\frac{1}{2}$ lemon, peeled
1 tbsp. cold-pressed oil (optional)
1 clove garlic (more or less, to taste)
2 basil leaves
$\frac{1}{2}$ tsp. sea salt
1 tbsp. wheat germ, raw (optional)
$\frac{1}{2}$ tsp. kelp (optional)
splash of vinegar (try red wine)
$\frac{1}{2}$ to 1 cup cold water (to the consistency you want)

Pepper Pot

5 to 6 green peppers
2 cups milk
1 tsp. sea salt

You can thicken the soup by using half and half instead of milk, or just drink as a juice by using water instead of the milk, if desired. If using without any dairy products, try a few drops of lemon juice with the water.

Cold Cucumber Soup

If you suspect the cucumber skins have been waxed, by all means peel them. Otherwise, if they're home-grown or unwaxed, mix them peel and all.

1 pound cucumbers (many people prefer Kirby cukes)
1/2 cup plain yogurt
1/2 tsp. sea salt
dried dill
dash of nutmeg

Party Dips and Spreads

Of course, we still need to eat foods in a variety of textures, and whole grain and vegetable fiber is very important. Why not try these recipes for dips that you can make in an instant in your juicer, and spread on whole grain breads, crackers, or use to dip young Romaine lettuce leaves and other veggies in? Besides being tasty and nutritious (because you make them fresh right before serving, and use the most wholesome ingredients), the ease of preparation when you have your own juicer makes these unusual dips just perfect for impromptu entertaining.

And many parents find that kids who turn their

Delicious Recipes to Try

noses up at cooked veggies just love eating them raw as finger foods—especially when they can scoop up lots of delicious dip along with the peppers, celery, broccoli, cucumbers, cauliflower, carrots or crunchy crackers and pita bread.

Because juicers are different, you need to get to know how yours operates. Take care to run your juicer or food processor just enough to blend the ingredients (in some cases, this may be only a matter of seconds), or strain as directed for a thicker dip. Otherwise, you'll end up with a soup!

Many of these dips use plain yogurt as a base—if you make your own, so much the better!

Yogurt Veggie Dip

1 cucumber (unpeeled)
½ green bell pepper
1 or 2 scallions (to taste)
1 tsp. kelp
1 clove garlic, peeled
pinch of thyme
½ tsp. fennel seeds
½ cup plain yogurt

Juice all of the above except the yogurt, then fold into the yogurt. Serve with fresh sprouts and an appetizing array of vegetables and crisp breads for dipping.

Cheese and Cukes

¹/₄ cup sour cream or plain yogurt
¹/₂ tsp. sea salt
1 tbsp. lemon juice
¹/₂ cup onion
1 large lettuce leaf
1 large cucumber
1 hard-boiled egg, peeled
1 ¹/₂ cups cottage cheese
1 tsp. fresh pepper or red pepper flakes

Mix all the ingredients together for about 10 seconds. Then enjoy!

Super-C Pepper Dip

Fresh, ripe peppers are very high in vitamin C—surpassing even oranges ands other citrus. Use green or red peppers or both, although the sweet red ones are tops in vitamin A content.

1 pound green and red sweet peppers
1 tsp. kelp
¹/₂ tsp. dill or sea salt

Juice the works for a refreshing drink, or, to prepare as a dip, juice the peppers first and strain them. Save the nutrient-rich liquid to drink or for soup later. Mix the kelp and salt into the mashed peppers and serve.

Zippy Zucchini Dip

¹/₂ pound zucchini
¹/₂ tsp. dill, sea or garlic salt

Juice, then strain extra liquid out before dipping.

Delicious Recipes to Try

The following dips use avocados, which will turn brown or gray if not used immediately. Cover the dip with waxed paper (right on the surface), with mayonnaise, extra lemon juice, or sour cream to hold until serving (smooth sour cream and mayonnaise over to coat completely). Or, mix ½ tsp. ascorbic acid (vitamin C) powder in to prevent it from turning color too soon.

Guacamole (Avocado Dip)

You must use soft avocados, but don't let them go brown first.

1 large or 2 small lemons, peeled and pitted
1 large, ripe avocado, split, pitted and peeled
1 tbsp. cold-pressed safflower or sunflower oil
2 to 3 cloves of garlic, peeled
1 small onion, peeled and with the root end cut off
1 small, ripe tomato
¼ tsp. sea salt
dash of fresh pepper or red pepper flakes (spicier)
2 tsp. wheat germ, raw
¼ tsp. kelp (optional)

Juice it up then serve immediately with soft flour or corn tortillas, corn chips, or over nachos.

Avocado Dip Too

2 ripe, peeled and pitted avocados
1 tbsp. lemon juice
2 tsp. hot taco sauce or tabasco
1 tbsp. onion
dash of pepper
$1/2$ tsp. sea salt or garlic salt
$1/2$ cup sour cream or plain yogurt
1 small, ripe tomato (optional)
4 slices crisp, crumbled bacon (optional)

Juice all ingredients at low speed to combine, or, add all but the bacon and use this as a garnish for the top when serving.

Nacho Man's Avocado, Bean and Cheese Dip

1 ripe, peeled and pitted avocado
1 tsp. lemon juice
1 8-oz. package cream cheese or tofu
1 16-oz. can of kidney beans
2 tomatoes, diced
4 scallions, chopped
1 cup cheddar cheese, grated or cubed
$1/2$ cup sliced black olives

Mix the first three ingredients in the juicer. Spread in a 9-inch pie plate. Rinse juicer. Drain kidney beans and puree in juicer. Spread bean mixture over avocado mix. Layer tomatoes and onions on top, then grated cheese (or mix cubes in juicer). Top with black olives and serve with fried tortillas or corn chips.

Delicious Recipes to Try

Eggplant Dip

The Lebanese call this tasty treat *baba ghannouj*. Whatever else you call it, you'll call it delicious.

2 large eggplants
2 lemons, peeled
2 tbsp. cold-pressed sunflower, safflower, or other
  vegetable oil
1 tsp. sea salt
2 to 3 cloves garlic, peeled

Trim and split the eggplants lengthwise, then lay face down on a baking sheet. Bake at 400 F. for about 40 minutes, or until the skin is crisp. Cool when done. Scrape the soft flesh out of the vegetable skin and mash, blend or juice with the lemons. Add the oil, salt and garlic and mix until of creamy consistency. Serve on pita toast, with raw cauliflower or cucumber or other crudites.

Tahini (Roasted Sesame Seeds) Butter

$1/2$ cup roasted sesame seeds
1 $1/3$ cup butter, slightly soft
2 oz. lemon juice
4 tsp. soy or tamari sauce

After mixing, chill slightly. Serve slightly soft on sandwiches, fancy crackers, or pita bread.

Cheesy Tomato Dip

8-oz. can of tomato sauce, or 6-8 ripe plum tomatoes
dash of fresh-ground pepper
4 oz. blue cheese
3 oz. cream cheese
¾ cup American or mild cheddar cheese

Mix in juicer until creamy and well-blended. Serve with fancy crackers, pita toasts or crisp breads.

Tasty Nut Butters

Check the instructions that came with your juicer to make sure your machine can handle these. The processing time can be a number of minutes to get the butter to the desired smoothness and consistency, causing some machines to run hot.

Cashew Butter

2 12-oz. cans or jars of cashews, salted or unsalted

Mix as directed for your machine. A splash or two of vegetable oil lends more smoothness. Salt to taste, if desired.

Peanut Butter

2 12-oz. cans or jars of peanuts, salted or unsalted
¼ cup peanut oil (if you are using dry-roasted peanuts)

Process as directed. Salt to taste, if desired.

Delicious Recipes to Try

Almond Butter

24 oz. toasted almonds, salted or unsalted
$^1/_4$-$^1/_2$ cup cold-pressed safflower or sunflower oil
salt to taste

Pecan Chutney

1 cup shelled pecans
3 oz. mango chutney
1 cup unsalted butter, slightly softened

Holiday Fare

Thanksgiving Cranberry Relish

2 cups firm cranberries
2 oranges, peeled and pitted
2 red apples, cored
$^1/_2$-1 cup sugar or honey (to taste)

Process to relish consistency. Some people like to include a bit of the orange peel for the color and texture it adds. Refrigerate a few hours before serving. This can also be made ahead of time and frozen. Add a dash of cinnamon or nutmeg if desired, or a splash of fruit liqueur.

CARLSON WADE is a well-known medical reporter with close to 40 books in the field of natural healing to his credit. His articles have appeared in many leading magazines and newspapers throughout the country, and his works have been translated into French, Spanish, German and Japanese. He makes frequent radio and television as well as personal appearances and is an accredited member of the American Medical Writers Association.